A SIMPLE BOOK
OF STRENGTH

TIM ANDERSON

CONTENTS

PREFACE

"It feels good to feel good."
- me

It's sad to say it, but that could be one of the biggest epiphanies I've ever had. It does feel good to feel good. Just recover from an injury or sickness; that mystery will be forever solved.

But do you know what makes you feel good or helps you overcome sickness?

Strength!

It feels good to be strong.

Having strength in your whole being- your body, mind, and soul- just makes everything better. When you have strength, life just seems easier and brighter. That's because when you have strength, YOU are better and more capable than you otherwise would be.

It feels good to be strong.

Having strength enables you to give your strength away and make the world a better, easier place to be. Think about this for a moment.

When you are weak, when you are sick, when you are injured, where do your thoughts go? What do they revolve around? Most of the time, you are self-absorbed. Your thoughts spiral around your condition, your predicament, and your inabilities. You cannot feel good when consumed with yourself due to limitations. Instead, you feel stuck or trapped and are not free from your mind. When you are not free from your mind, you do not make the world a better place because you cannot freely give yourself to the world.

But when you are strong and feel good, how self-absorbed are you? Typically, you're not self-absorbed because you are free from limitations and lack. Having strength is the absence of limitations. When you don't have limitations, you don't have self-obsessions; instead, you have vision. You can "see" others and naturally want to offer yourself to others.

Having strength makes the world better because it flows from you to those around you. It bolsters others. Maybe you smile at a stranger, take the grocery cart back to the store for a shopper, or listen to a friend struggling with a severe life change. Strength allows you to be there for the world, support it, comfort it, and carry it. And that feels good.

Yes, it feels good to feel good. But the truth is that it feels good to do good. And the ability to freely be and do good comes from having strength from being free from physical, mental, and emotional limitations.

It feels good to do good.

That's what this book is about. Removing our limitations allows us to express the strength we have all been given. You are designed to be strong.

Everything about your nervous system highlights this fact. This can only mean you are designed to feel good. I'll go a step further and say you are designed to feel amazing.

I hope you discover your strength and learn what it is like to feel amazing. Because, believe it or not, it feels good to feel amazing.

INTRODUCTION

"Strength is a skill."
- Pavel Tsatsouline

Strength is a skill, but is also so much more than that. It's an expression of who you are and what is inside you. It's something you were born to have. It's something you were made to be.

Strength has different qualities; like any skill, it can be cultivated differently. But like an expression, strength has gradients and can be seen as a spectrum.

Each of us has a level of strength we can express, a level that we have access to. And each of us has a level of strength potential - one that most of us will never tap into. This book aims to help you tap into your strength potential to help you gain access to the strength inside of you.

You have physical strength. You have mental strength. You have the strength of discipline. You have the strength of choice.

You have the strength of character. None of these are separate. They are all one. They are all you.

There are many training programs to be found here, and many ways to practice your strength. But there may also be new ways to see and think about strength. This book is about training and moving with purpose to unlock your strength as an expression, not necessarily as a skill of display. Although unencumbered expression is quite the skill to master.

If you want to practice the skill of strength training in pursuit of bodybuilding, powerlifting, or Olympic lifting, this book may not be for you. But if you want to perfect the expression of your strength, to have unfettered access to it in your day-to-day life, this may be what you are looking for.

Strength is your essence.

Let it out.

"You are much stronger than you think you are. Trust me."
- Absolute All-Star Superman

REALITY AND A DISCLAIMER

Exercise has risks associated with it. Research shows that it can lead to being stronger, healthier, and happier. However, it can also lead to injuries or even death. It happens. You should also know that doing nothing also has risks associated with it. Research shows that being sedentary can lead to sickness, weakness, frailty, depression, and anxiety. It can also make you more injury-prone and hasten your destination towards death. It happens.

Before engaging in any exercise program, consult your trusted family physician. But also, before you engage in any sedentary lifestyle, you should also consult with your trusted family physician.

"Every man dies, but not every man really lives."
- William Wallace, Braveheart

THE STRUGGLE IS REAL

"Where there is no struggle, there is no strength."
- Oprah Winfrey

You were born through struggle. A baby passing through the birth canal is no easy task for the mother or the child. Then there is the struggle of being abruptly presented with the outside world. We go from pitch dark, warm, and cozy to insanely bright, cold, and loud.

This struggle helps prepare us for life out in the world. Our bodies are made to "rise to the occasion." If the baby responds appropriately with vigor (good color, good vitals, good lungs), he expresses his strength. If the baby doesn't respond appropriately, or if there was too much trauma during birth, he may have a low Apgar score and will likely need some additional attention, love, and care, possibly including resuscitation, to assist in rekindling and releasing his strength.

After birth, the real struggle begins as the baby begins its fight against gravity. This is the struggle that builds the brain and ties the entire body together. As the baby learns to balance its overly large head and keep it level with the horizon, it builds amazing physical strength and endurance, eventually pulling itself up on two feet.

By the way, the helplessness of a human baby combined with its ingrained developmental reflexes and the peculiarly large head that contains its gravitational detection system (the vestibular system) is an ingenious design. The struggle through this helplessness that seeks to manage and control the enormity of the human head gives birth to amazing strength. It's not just thumbs and being bipedal that set us apart from all the other animals found in nature. It's also the design of the proportions in which we are born. We were literally born to be strong.

We were literally born to be strong.

Anyway, the struggle against gravity builds, harnesses, and releases the baby's strength for full expression. Also, as a developing child has learned very few fears from the world, it has very few limiters placed on its body, until it accrues them.

The point is, your entire life is a series of moments and struggles that yield opportunities for you to build and express your strength. Strength is built and cultivated through challenge. But strength is expressed through freedom.

We all have enormous strength potential, but not all of us have access to our strength. As an expression, strength can be governed by the nervous system. If the brain does not feel it is safe to express the body's strength, it will limit that expression.

The brain is an organ of inhibition and is, therefore, the gatekeeper to our strength. In order to have access to our strength potential, the brain has to feel safe enough about the body's condition to grant that access. After all, it doesn't want us to jeopardize the health of the vehicle that ensures its survival.

This is where struggle comes in. Struggle, or challenge, is the key to releasing our strength. It gives us practice in learning our barriers, developing our responses, and summoning our resources. Again, our bodies are made to rise to the occasion, and we do this through a natural series of trials that we experience in our day-to-day lives. Or at least we should.

But many of our lives in today's world are very comfortable. We don't necessarily face day-to-day challenges that help ensure the presence and availability of our strength. This is why many of us need to purposefully practice being uncomfortable - we need to provide a stimulus, a challenge, to the body that asks the body to adapt in strength.

Continual dosages of discomfort build strength and prepare the brain for granting access to our strength. If the brain knows we can handle the strain and knows we are not foreigners to discomfort, it will feel safe to grant us access to our strength when we want it. After all, we will have prepared the body to express it.

There are exceptions and occasions of full access to unfettered strength, but they are rare. The exceptions are powerful, though, in that they support the truth that you have all the strength you could ever hope or imagine to have in your body right now. I'm talking about supernatural expressions of strength in emergencies.

Grandma Strong

We've all heard the stories. Somehow, in a miracle display of strength, a seemingly old and frail grandma picks a car up off of her grandchild. Things like this have and do happen.

I recently saw a news story on TV about a young teenage girl lifting a car off of her dad's chest. He had been working underneath his car when the jack failed. The car crashed down, pinning him underneath. Being compressed, he couldn't cry for help. Fortunately, his daughter came to the garage looking for him and noticed he was being crushed. Without THINKING, she deadlifted the car up off his chest and moved it to the side. She may have weighed about 130 pounds. The car probably weighed around 3000 pounds.

She was just an average teenager. She was not a performing strongman, and she had not been practicing the skills of strength. And yet, she expressed the amount of strength that powerlifters and performing strongmen dream about and train to have. She had been given full access to her strength and tapped into it through an emergency. At the speed of her nervous system recognizing the threat, her autonomic nervous system dumped an adrenaline cocktail powerful enough to block rationality and unlock all of her physical inhibitions; without thought or hesitation, she picked up a car off of her dad's chest and saved his life.

It's amazing. And it's a beautiful display of the strength and potential in each and every one of us. Also, just as amazing, the girl was unhurt. She suffered no injuries from moving that car - no tears, no breaks.

How can this happen? Was the girl a gym rat? Had she spent her life practicing strength training and the deadlift? No. She was acting to save her father, whom she loved. She had no other options but action. And she took it.

She didn't warm up. She didn't think her way through it. She didn't use physics, levers, and mechanical advantages. She grabbed underneath the car and lifted it with her unbridled strength.

Sometimes, in the right scenario (like an emergency), we can tap into our full potential for strength expression. This is rare, but it does happen.

To be 100% open, this girl didn't tap into her full strength potential. That would have hurt her. But she did tap into what she needed. And that's the point: we all have ALL the strength that we need stored inside us.

And more.

Did you know that people who have suffered from electric shock have been known to break their own bones and dislocate their own joints? Yep, the body's muscles have enough strength to break the bones they are connected to, rip the tendons, and dislocate the joints of those bones. This strength is sometimes seen when electricity commandeers the full contractile strength of muscles.

> **We all have ALL the strength that we need stored inside us.**

By the way, it should be understood that when electrocution happens, and the muscles break bones, this is not isolated to muscle-bound individuals. This happens with regular, non-muscle-bound people, though unfortunate people. Please know that I'm not making light of electrocutions but merely trying to illustrate the strength potential in your body.

Again, you have more than enough strength in your body to do amazing things or to simply live the life you want to live.

Finding Comfort in Struggle with Your RPE

The Rate of Perceived Exertion is a subjective self-measuring scale used to determine effort level or challenge level on a scale of 1 to 10 or 0 to 10 for those who want more choices. Still, there is an RPE scale from 6 to 20 for those wanting even more classification choices. As I think a scale that runs from 6 to 20 is just a bit weird, I'll stick with the 1 to 10 scale for the purposes of this book. Anyway, the RPE is a way to measure your struggle or how hard you think you are working.

Strength is born through struggle. This is Nature's design. This is why a baby animal must work its own way out of an egg. This boosts its chance of survival. From the lens of "Survival of the fittest," it is the "fittest" who have adapted well through struggle.

From a strength training perspective, data suggests that growth happens in the struggle zone of 70-80% of max effort or load. For example, if the absolute most a person can military press overhead is 100 pounds, practicing the

Strength is born through struggle.

military press with 70 pounds is where they will likely make their greatest gains in strength. The 70 pounds should be a challenging amount of weight that allows them to successfully perform the movement for their prescribed number of attempts. It requires an effort that can become uncomfortable. Being uncomfortable but successful is where the growth of strength happens.

ODDVAR HOLTEN DIAGRAM

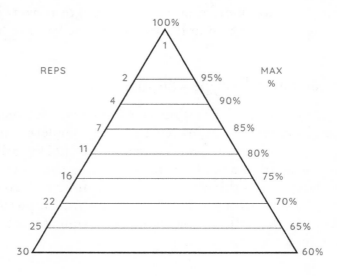

Here is the Oddvar Holten Diagram. I'm only presenting this for those wanting to know things or have data. This information is not needed for the purposes of this book, but it may broaden your understanding of the "Struggle Zone" of the 70% - 80% of max effort that I mentioned above.

The diagram shows the relationship between maximum strength and relative muscular endurance. It's a useful scale to help determine your desired or needed training load percentage. While the diagram may not be 100% accurate for you, it can help get you in the ballpark of where you need to be. Or at least it can help you better understand where you are in your training loads.

The Oddvar Holten Diagram can be used to determine the desired training percentage and repetition range if the load of the one-repetition max is known, or it can be used in reverse to estimate what one's one-repetition max (or desired training repetition range and load) by lifting a weight for as many reps as possible.

For example, if Billy can only bench press 100 pounds. The curve shows us that 70% of Billy's training load would be 70 pounds, and with 70 pounds, Billy can likely perform 22 straight presses.

Or, let's imagine that Billy can bench press 70 pounds 20 times. If we look at the diagram, we can see that Billy is likely training with 70% of his one rep max. With some math, we can determine Billy's 85% training load and rep range.

70 pounds = 70%X

X= 70 pounds / 0.7

X = 100 (Billy's max)

100(.85) = 85 pounds. Looking at the diagram, Billy can likely press this 7 times before failure.

Again, this curve can be useful in determining and gauging your appropriately challenging training loads. An appropriate challenge is where the load, rep range or task creates a struggle, but you are successful in lifting or performing the task for the desired objectives. If you struggle with this diagram or with doing math, there is an app for that. In fact, there are several rep range calculators you can download on your phone.

Strength is cultivated through successful challenges or struggles.

Just remember, strength is cultivated through successful challenges or struggles.

Another way to determine challenging efforts that allow for success and growth is to use the Rate of Perceived Exertion scale (RPE) from 1 - 10. With the RPE, a 7 would be the 70% area of effort that causes discomfort. You could also call the RPE the Struggle Scale.

When it comes to building physical AND mental strength, struggling in the 5 to 8 range of the RPE on a scale of 10 is where progress is made. This is a great training range as this is the range that is often uncomfortable but doable.

And that's what we want. We want to train in the realm of uncomfortable but doable. The place where we are challenged but successful in our efforts.

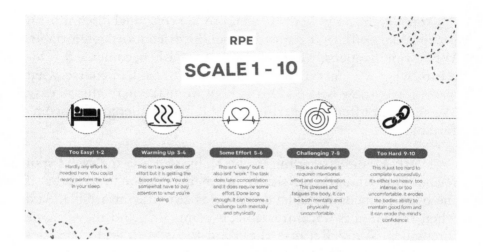

Layers of Strength

OK, there are layers and levels of strength. And as you know, strength can come and go and come again. At least, it can appear to.

Ultimately, strength is born in the nervous system.

When it comes to building and expressing neurological strength, it is showing up often in the window of discomfort that allows us to harness our strength to express it at will. If we show up often enough, our nervous system gets stronger and more efficient by creating strong neural pathways.

Strength is built through the body's desire to adapt to stressors.

But showing up often long enough also causes our tissues to get stronger through growth and adaptation. Muscles, tendons, fascia - these tissues are made bigger, thicker, and stronger through being exposed to repeated stress. This is how strength training works; it takes advantage of the body's desire to adapt.

Strength is built through the body's desire to adapt to stressors.

You see, the body wants to adapt to the continual discomfort it is being exposed to - it wants to make the discomfort comfortable. When this happens, what was once a 7 RPE becomes a 5. This means what was once a 10 may now be an 8. And, of course, what was a 5 may now be a 3. This is how we make hard things easy. We show up often and perform doable but challenging, uncomfortable tasks.

Working and struggling in the realm of a 7 is the sweet spot for building strength, physically and mentally. Don't forget that if the body is uncomfortable, the mind is also uncomfortable. And when the mind is uncomfortable, it complains, and the struggle intensifies. Why? Because the mind focuses on and magnifies what it perceives to be the irritant. And where the attention goes, everything else follows, including the body. Remember this: the body follows the head in physical form and creative thought.

Anyway, when you become comfortable with struggle, it is not just your body that is stronger; it's also your mind. Strengthening the mind is key to strengthening the body. Training wisely in struggle and discomfort is a great way to tame the mind, discipline it, and teach it how to let go of struggle. In other words, you can learn to accept discomfort.

When you know you can do hard things, and your mind is unscathed by discomfort, your body will follow the path of "I can." Confidence, "I can-ness," is a great way to remove neurological inhibition so that the body can freely express its strength.

Perhaps the biggest reason for the gain in strength and ease is that the brain wants balance. If we continually show up for a challenge, the brain will recruit resources to eliminate the challenge. The brain doesn't want to waste energy. It wants to secure energy. If we are learning a new skill, building strength, or being uncomfortable often, the brain will find a way to get the body efficient so that the struggle is less. In other words, the brain will make it so that the body adapts to the challenge to eliminate it or diminish the struggle.

Again, this happens through showing up often. It's much like a tree that starts growing toward the sun's direction - it adapts to get the resources it needs to flourish. The brain wants to secure survival and flourish in homeostasis, so it adapts the body to repetitive challenges in order to secure resources and achieve energy conservation. This is sometimes called the SAID principle: Specific Adaptation to Imposed Demand - basically, the body adapts to what it does.

This happens for *appropriate* challenges.

When the challenge is not appropriate or too little, there is no struggle or stimulus to adapt to. When the challenge is too great, like a 10 or a 10.5, or not doable, and the effort persists beyond logical reason, the body will likely get injured. When an injury occurs, the brain will send resources to heal and repair the body as best it can. At this point, the brain may also find ways to keep you from trying to challenge your body until it's ready to be challenged. The brain is not concerned with optimal performance in the presence of an injury but with healing. Pain signals, weakness, and limited range of motion are some of the inhibitors the brain places on the body during the healing process.

Injuries can have long-lasting effects on both the body and the mind. The nervous system can hold onto a "memory" of an injury. It may continue to try to protect the body through pain or weakness long after the injury has healed. Also, injuries result in compensatory movement patterns that may need to be unlearned or "reprogrammed." For example, a sprained ankle may result in a limp. When the ankle heals, the nervous system may still be running some of the "limp" programs because the stability and mobility of the ankle have not been reset and restored.

The nervous system can hold onto a "memory" of an injury.

Injuries also greatly affect the mind. You can't neglect the role of your thoughts and memories after an injury, either. They will likely also become performance inhibitors that you may need to heal from. Fear and fear of reinjury are powerful performance inhibitors.

The point is, when adding load or increasing the challenge, the challenge must be appropriate. This bears repeating 1000 times: a doable struggle, that's what we want. A doable struggle is a place that is just off the edge of discomfort. This is where huge strides can be made in releasing our strength potential - neurologically, physically, mentally, and emotionally.

Is Perceived Exertion Real Exertion?

Kind of.

Okay, so there is a potential issue with perceived exertion; it is perceived. This is where knowing oneself and honest assessments come into play.

Some people's perception meter may not be accurate. This is often due to a lack of experience in what they are doing or actually a lack of discomfort in their day-to-day lives. There are people who have never been exposed to hard tasks (manual labor or tasks at the edge of their capacity), and there are plenty of people who have no experience with strength training. If they don't know what a struggle is, they may have a very narrow comfort zone or be hypersensitive to slight discomfort.

But discomfort is discomfort. Even if their perception meter needs calibrating, if a person truly feels uncomfortable with a task or movement, YET they show up anyway in honest curiosity; they will experience growth of some kind in any of the possible areas for growth. They will gain more access to their strength because they challenge their comfort level. The key here is that they are being honest about their level of discomfort, and they are intent on exploring it. In other words, if a person starts where they are, with or without an accurate perception of their effort and discomfort levels, they can still make great strides in strength by showing up.

This is where an alternative RPE scale can come in handy - The Doable Scale, where understanding "doable but challenging" comes into play. It can help a person to qualify their effort. Converting the RPE to a Doable Scale can be helpful, and it can look like this:

easily doable, no challenge (1-4 RPE)

doable, but challenging (5-7 RPE)

barely doable (8-9 RPE)

not doable (10 RPE)

And yes, an RPE of 5 can be challenging. Especially if what is being done requires focus and control - this challenges the mind. Remember, we aren't just physical bodies; we are body, mind, and soul. There may be tasks or exercises that are physically an RPE of 5 but mentally a 7. Growth and progress can still be made here. It all depends on the purpose and intent of the training. And training should have a purpose. Ultimately though, that purpose should be to gain access to and freely express your strength.

The RPE and Doable Scale can be easy to calibrate and *less* subjective when we are dealing with concrete numbers like a prescribed number of sets and reps. Let's imagine that a set calls for 5 reps, and we were able to complete 5, but we know we could have completed 7, 2 more than needed. We are likely around an RPE of 7, or "Doable, but challenging." Here, we are using an appropriate load for the prescribed set.

If the set calls for 5 reps, but we could only do 3 reps, we are definitely at an RPE of 10, or "not doable." Here, we should lighten the load to be able to complete the prescribed set.

If the set calls for 5 reps, and we can do 10 reps with minor discomfort, we are around an RPE of 3 or 4, "easily doable." Here, we should increase the amount of weight used so that achieving 5 reps is a challenge.

Yes, it is still subjective, but with time and experience, you can learn your effort level fairly well. Really, you don't need to overthink it. When you are training, just be aware of where you are in your efforts. Are you being challenged? Did it make you uncomfortable? Were you successful in your task(s)? If the answer is "yes," you will grow and harness your strength.

Also, just know that when it comes to training, as in life, nothing is absolute. There will be days when you need to train at a 5, not a 7 or 8. Your body will tell you when those days are - if you listen to it and honor it. If you are not good at listening to your body, planning variations into your strength training can also be a great training practice.

And not to cause confusion, but every day does not need to be a day where you challenge yourself. Some days just need to be days where you show up. You can build a lot of strength by challenging yourself just two to three days a week. But you can learn to harness that strength by showing up on the other days.

Showing Up

"If it is important, do it every day."
- Dan Gable and Dan John

Showing up is really the key, especially if we are talking about neural efficiency and strength. We can actually show up enough and slide the scale of our RPE. This is why Dan John's Easy Strength is so effective; you show up every day and perform 5 exercises for 10 reps each. That's it. Most days are light, in the 3 to 5 range of the RPE (yes, most days are "easily doable"). Some days are a challenge, around a 7, maybe an 8. But all days are "Show Up" days.

Showing up builds neural strength in the patterns we are using. It creates very efficient neural pathways. Efficient neural pathways are strong pathways that don't use much excess energy. Showing up takes advantage of the "use it or lose it" principle, which can also be seen as the "use it to build it" or "use and keep it" principle.

This means if you show up enough, without training too intensely (in the 9 and 10 range) too often, you can create a strength that is always there, ready for you to tap into. At least in those patterns, you've been showing up for. If you choose the right patterns, you will find great carryover in your strength out in the "real world," and you can live your life well.

Showing up also creates familiarity in your nervous system. When a pattern is familiar to the nervous system, there is little cause for concern as the pattern is not seen as a threat or something that should be inhibited. Familiar, efficient neural pathways are not inhibited by the nervous system or the mind, and they are freer to express the body's strength, speed, and power. This is one reason why training and practice are so important for the qualities we want to express. When the body is prepared through repetition, freedom of expression results.

Again, it's the "use it and keep it" principle, but it starts as the "use it and build it" principle. We are simply taking advantage of our nervous system's plasticity (the flexible malleability) through consistent engagement. This gives us access to uninhibited movements and expressions and keeps us prepared for life (again, if we practice the right patterns) because we will not lose what we've been showing up for.

Keep this in mind. There is a diminishing return for how hard we train and how strong we can get; training too hard will only result in losing strength, performance, and possible injuries. But there is no diminishing return for intelligently showing up; we can keep most of the strength we've built with consistent effort through neural efficiency and strong neural pathways.

And remember, we each have far more strength in our bodies than we will ever need. But what we do need is access to that strength. Showing up often and intelligently gives us access to that strength; it allows us the freedom of expression.

Showing Up and the RPE

You may be wondering, wait, does training in a level of challenge or discomfort build strength, or does showing up often build strength?

Yes.

They both build strength. Showing up builds strength in your nervous system. Training through challenge and discomfort builds strength in your muscles, tendons, and fascia. But strength is larger than physical expression. Showing up often also strengthens the mind through discipline and routine. Successfully training in challenge and discomfort builds strength and confidence in the mind. A disciplined, confident mind also removes inhibitions from the body's expressions. In other words, a strong mind can give you access to a strong body, *and* physical training can help you build a stronger mind. Strength in one area can lead to strength in all other areas.

But let's talk a little more about showing up and the RPE. We want to train intelligently and get the most out of our bodies so we can live our lives as uninhibited as possible. This means looking for the minimum effective dose of discomfort/challenge/

training may be wise. As I stated above, showing up and training in discomfort, around 7 or 8, may only need to be done twice to thrice a week, depending on what you are doing.

Showing up every day and training at a 7 or 8 without letting the body adequately recover will most likely lead to overtraining and injury. At the right dose or frequency, the right challenge or effort needs to be recovered from. Recovery is where growth is going to be found. Not allowing for recovery, always tapping into our sub-maximal efforts, will erode our strength gains and the health of our tissues. In other words, recovery is integral to strength training and expression.

Training around an RPE of 7 or 8 for two to three days a week while showing up every other day and training in an RPE of 3 to 5 can allow for recovery and growth. Showing up and practicing the right movement patterns at lower intensities can even accelerate the recovery process, allowing for optimal growth and expression.

I know this can get confusing, but that's why we are here.

We are made to move. In fact, we are designed to move a lot. In other words, we were not built for a sedentary life. Training for an hour out of one day, two to three days a week, is still living a sedentary life. I would argue that training one hour out of the day and being sedentary for the rest of your waking hours is still living a sedentary life. Anyway, It is the daily engagement of movement that gives us access to being able to keep engaging *daily*. Not engaging in our daily movement design opens the door to not having full access to our performance potential and freedom of expression.

Don't get me wrong, you can build strength and size from training with heavy loads or submaximally intense efforts only two to three days per week, but if you do nothing else the other four to five days a week, you'll likely be more limited in your ability to express your strength and performance potential. You may get stronger and bigger, but you'll likely be limited in your strength expression outside the weight room. Not only that but if you're living a mostly sedentary life but training hard or heavy for two to three days a week for an hour at a time, you're really not improving your health all that much. You may even be taxing it more.

Don't miss that point. Strength is not health; health doesn't come from heavy strength training or "working out" two to three hours a week. Health comes from using your body and moving often, how it was designed to be used and moved. Health comes from showing up every day.

If you only care about weight room performance, then training hard and heavy a few hours a week may be enough for you. But if you care about your life performance and your health, showing up daily or almost daily at lower intensity levels sprinkled around your more intense training days can give you a broader foundation of strength AND health that will serve you far more in life.

All of that to say, your purpose - your why - in training matters. If you want to express your full potential and be as uninhibited as possible, daily engagement in moving will serve you well. Challenging yourself with more intensity (6 to 8 RPE) two to three days a week and showing up in curiosity and exploration (3 to 5 RPE) the rest of the week is a great way to gain access to your strength. This can give you the best of everything: uninhibited neural, physical, and mental strength that allows you to live your life to your full potential.

I'll provide some examples of what this may look like later in the book. For now, just understand what an RPE is and how to gauge your effort.

Now, to really muddy up the whole thing. If this is all too much to take in, just show up every day or as much as you can and aim for the middle. Pretend you're Goldilocks and find that "just right" effort level (about a 5 RPE). For Goldilocks, life was found in the middle of the extremes. I know, I was talking about 7 to 8 RPEs and growth and recovery and all of that. But adaptation to imposed demand is still an adaptation. If you always hit the middle (RPE of 5), the middle gets ridiculously easy to hit, meaning you are stronger, and you're

Show up often and explore challenging your strength through practice.

sliding your RPE further to the right, creating a new middle. When 5's become 3s, 7s become 5s. Don't overthink this - show up often and explore challenging your strength through practice.

STRENGTH PRACTICE VS
STRENGTH PUNISHMENT

This is a public service announcement:

If you exercise, move, train, or whatever, it should be a joyful practice and not a form of punishment.

Practice your strength. Don't punish yourself in pursuit of it. That's almost as weird as destroying your house frantically looking for your car keys while you have them in your closed hand the whole time. You already have what you think you don't, and there is no need to punish yourself to enjoy it. In fact, if you punish yourself in the name of strength training, you will likely not be able to enjoy your strength at all.

If you are of the mindset that strength training should be hard, that you need to vomit at the end of every practice, that someone needs to stand over you and spray you with saliva as they yell obscenities at you, then you will likely not be able to enjoy your strength. Instead, you may inhibit it even more. Not to mention, you'll likely make yourself miserable and set yourself up for a life of failed attempts to be fit, strong, and healthy.

I'm kind of talking about the "No Pain, No Gain" mindset, but this is bigger than that. First of all, pain is a threat to your nervous system. Pain is one of the fastest ways to inhibit your strength. Not to mention, physical pain is most likely your body's polite way of asking you to stop hurting it. If you've ever been injured by pushing through pain, you know you've had that thought, "I should have listened to my body."

This may be a great time to point out that there is a difference between discomfort and pain. Discomfort is simply being uncomfortable. Pain is pain; it hurts. Strength and growth are born out of challenge. But pain gives birth to depression, anxiety, and injury.

Pain is one of the fastest ways to inhibit your strength.

You can curiously and joyfully approach discomfort. This is your practice. But don't blindly train in pain for pain. This is your punishment. At best, it will lead to "lessons learned," but it can also lead to much more misery than you should have to try to overcome.

Here is where I differ from many people in the strength world. I am a proponent of only training and practicing movements that bring you joy or satisfy your curiosity. I'm not a fan of training movements that you hate to do.

The argument can be made that doing movements you hate to do can benefit you. They can strengthen areas you need to focus on. Sure, that may be so, but it's like eating. I know broccoli can be good for me. It has vitamins and minerals that could make my body healthier. But I'm not going to eat broccoli because I simply do not enjoy broccoli. Other things I can eat will give me those same vitamins and minerals. And by not eating broccoli, I am happier as I enjoy the foods I eat.

Similarly, if you hate doing kettlebell swings, don't do them. There are other movements you can do that will give you the same strength and athleticism that kettlebell swings could give you. Participating in movements you don't like will result in you just "checking the box" to get through it. This is not practice; it's punishment. It can even become survival as you are just trying to get through it. There is no longevity in this. Even if there is, what's the point if you're miserable? Not to mention, just checking the box on a movement you are trying to survive can set you up for a physical injury.

But practicing the movements you enjoy will give you training longevity. It will also allow you to become more creative and curious, begging your focus and attention as you practice. In turn, the practice will nourish your soul along with your body. You will feel better through practicing with movements you enjoy.

Don't punish yourself. If you like broccoli, eat it. If you don't, eat something else that can give you the same benefits. Likewise, if you like kettlebell swings, do them. If you don't, explore other movements like hill sprints, skipping, or the power clean. You get the idea.

Approaching strength through joy and curiosity will give you access to more strength expression because no dread is attached to it. Dread is a threat and an expression dampener. It sets you up for weakness, not strength.

Discipline

You should also be aware of the Discipline Trap. Discipline can be your friend if you use it wisely. But it can also be your taskmaster if you let it use you.

Showing up to train every day because you *want* to can lead to wonderful practice sessions. Showing up to train every day because you *have* to can lead to miserable punishment sessions.

If you have discipline, use it with discernment. Listen to your body and read your situation. It may be best to heed if you want to train but your body is giving you a contrary message. You will not lose strength by abstaining from training for a day or three if your body tells you to do so. However, if you ignore your body, you could miss several training days if you create an injury.

This is really about flexibility and rigidity. If you have discipline, you are better off having an open, flexible discipline. An example of this may be being mentally committed to showing up every day but open enough to allow life to force you to call an audible. Whether the audible means skipping the day, training later in the day, or changing the exercises you had planned for the day - it's simply about being open to pivot as needed. This is flexibility, and it can serve you well.

A rigid discipline, on the other hand, is not so accommodating. It's closed-minded and blind due to the tasks at hand. An example of this would be being determined to show up every day even if you're sick with the flu - you will train no matter what. Or, it could be *come hell or high water*, Monday is Chest day, dammit, even if your shoulder is telling you not to bench press. Rigid discipline is a trap of woes. It owns you, and it can lead you to much pain and suffering.

Be flexible. This means if you're on vacation with your family, you don't have to look for the nearest gym. It's okay to take a break and spend time with your family. One day, you will likely regret all those times when you left them for one to three hours to train while on vacation. You will miss moments and memories because your discipline overrides your reason. I made this mistake far too many times when I was younger and when my kids were younger. I have nothing to show for it but the things I missed out on. There was no glory to be found by leaving them to go train. Not to mention that I didn't even need any equipment to train with in order to reveal my strength, and I

Be flexible.

didn't need to leave my family to train at all - but I didn't know that then, or I was too caught up in my discipline to see the truth.

Let's actually talk about strength for a second.

Strength comes in many forms. Sometimes, it can take more strength to abstain from training than it takes to train. Strength can be found in saying "no," walking away from something, or even quitting something. It pays to exercise that type of strength as well.

Exercise your judgment and intellect, and build them up. Don't be a slave to discipline or routine. Be in charge of your reasons for training or not training. Don't let discipline mask your obsession and insecurities, but do use discipline to protect your desire to express and experience your strength.

Strength is not about blindly showing up to check a box for a perfect attendance award that no one cares about. This will not make your life any better. I'm sorry, but It just won't.

Strength training should be about showing up to explore and enjoy the body that you have and the skills you want to develop. It's about being able to live your life in full expression with the people you care about. This not only makes your life better, it makes your life awesome.

Guilt

Speaking of discipline, you also need to be aware of guilt. Guilt is almost always a lie meant to control you. Do not feel guilty if you choose to miss a training session. Do not feel guilty if you *have to* miss a training session. The guilt comes from a fear inside of you, and it is a lie.

You have to give life permission to happen. Because whether you like it or not, whether you plan for it or not, life does and will happen. And that needs to be okay. There is no need to feel guilty over a missed training session, or anything else for that matter.

Guilt is a self-generated threat. Meaning you create guilt through whatever thoughts your brain comes up with. The purpose of the guilt is to break you into submission, to coerce you, or to belittle you.

Guilt is a self-generated threat. I know you generate it, and it aims to inflict harm on yourself. Yes, it seems weird, but the ego makes interesting lies sometimes. You need to be aware of these lies so that you don't allow guilt to threaten your freedom because that's what it does.

Again, guilt is a threat, so naturally, your nervous system will respond to the threat. Your emotions will swing negatively, your thoughts will take on a negative slant, your muscles will be filled with tension, and all of your body's systems will shift into survival mode. Guilt is a huge performance limiter, an expression dampener, and a thief of strength.

Accepting guilt is self-punishment. If you force yourself to train or do anything out of guilt, you are punishing yourself and, therefore, limiting your strength.

All of this is to say, allow life to happen without accepting the blame. Let whatever it is go and move on. If you miss a training session, it's going to be ok. You've not ruined or jeopardized anything. You've got your whole life to explore, practice, and express your strength. Enjoy it.

You are not guilty. Allowing life to happen is a form of strength training as well. It takes and builds immense strength.

THE TRUTH ABOUT STRENGTH

Strength is multifaceted. It is built layer upon layer and by thread intertwined with thread. It permeates through and flows from ALL of you. It is the pure expression of the dance between body, mind, and soul.

Strength has many qualities. It can be gentle, explosive, slow, fast, enduring, bursting, smooth, and fluid. It can be seen as drive, grit, passion, hope, *Strength is your essence.* tenacity, patience, confidence, stillness, and silence. It is all of these things and so much more.

Essentially, strength is your essence.

It's what you were meant to express all of your life. It's your wellspring. It's who you are.

But that's a deep notion, so let's start here first:

The Body

"A cord of three strands is not easily broken."
- Ecclesiastes 4:12, CSB

Strength begins in the body with the nervous system. Before you were born, your nervous system had a series of programs, reflexes, and movement patterns designed to weave everything about you together. These patterns and reflexes weren't just intended to make your muscles stronger and your movements smoother; they were intended to continue to build and develop all the systems in your body, literally building you from the inside out.

Strength builds upon itself.

When you carried out these patterns as a child, you constructed a healthy, strong, and efficient nervous system. The stronger your nervous system became, the stronger your body grew in size, strength, and capability.

Those reflexes and patterns you were born with developed your nervous system, giving you more access to your body. You developed stability, mobility, control, coordination, rhythm, and, ultimately, finesse.

The more you gained access, the more you could express through movement. These new expressions, in turn, continue to build your nervous system. Again, strength begets strength.

There were some essential components of those pre-programmed reflexes and patterns. Indeed, those essential components were to be woven into and throughout all the movements you would ever make in your entire lifetime. These are the three components of strength, the three things you were always intended to do to freely express your strength potential:

Breathe with an uninhibited diaphragm.

Activate your vestibular system through movement and having full control of your head.

Engage in your full gait pattern.

These three things are woven throughout the entire developmental sequence of a child. These three things are the foundation of your body's ability to move with freedom and strength. These three things are also the foundation of you - who you are, how you feel, and how you think.

You could even look at these three things as three keys. They are the keys to the kingdom of *you*.

Breathing with an Uninhibited Diaphragm

As far as the body's ability to express strength goes, strength starts here. An uninhibited diaphragm is the core, or the epicenter, of strength.

What is an uninhibited diaphragm?

It is the diaphragm you were born with, the jellyfish-like muscle that fills your lungs from the bottom to the top and from the back to the front. The muscle that descends into the abdominal cavity, displacing the organs as it makes room for the lungs to expand. It's the muscle that stabilizes and protects the spine as it moves. It's also the muscle that is neurologically connected to the other stabilizers in the center of the body, like the pelvic floor, the psoas, the transverse abdominis, and all the other spinal stabilizers.

When the diaphragm is uninhibited, the center of the body *is* strong because all the other spinal stabilizers and deep core muscles are fluidly working together in cooperation. This protects the spine and allows you to generate immense force and power. It also tells your brain that your body is ready and able to express that power. When the diaphragm is not inhibited, the brain feels safe, and this safety allows for full expressive potential.

You must understand your brain is always scanning your body, looking for strength. When the brain receives the information it is looking for when it sees that every member, every pattern, and every messenger is securely connected and transmitting "safe" information, "strong" information, the brain allows the body to express itself freely. If the brain does not detect the signals, connections, and operations of strength, it does not feel safe, and it will inhibit the body's ability to express itself. It makes things tight, sends pain signals, it dampens strength expression and greatly limits force production.

Breathing properly with an uninhibited diaphragm sends the one message the brain seeks: "I am strong." It is essentially what the Old Testament talks about when it instructs a warrior to "Gird up your loins." It is strengthening yourself in your very center, preparing yourself for action, durability, and power. Strength is the original design of breath. What I mean is strength comes from breath.

How you breathe determines every minute thing about your body, your mind, and your emotions. It is the bedrock of who you are. Your breath either allows for the expression of strength or invites fear and weakness to fill your mind and body. Yes, that is true.

Strength comes from breath.

If you want to be strong and express your strength, you must breathe as you were designed to.

The design of your breath looks like this:

Breathe nasally with your tongue resting against the roof of your mouth behind your front teeth. Allow your diaphragm to descend down in a 360° fashion, expanding not only your belly but your ribs, your sides, and your back. Allow your lungs to be filled and emptied slowly. The breath is meant to be long and full, not short, shallow, and incomplete.

This is the way you were born breathing. This is the way you are meant to breathe. This is the beginning of strength.

Vestibular System Powers, Activate!

As I mentioned earlier in the book, one of the miracles of the human body is found in the proportions we are born with. Being able to gain control of a watermelon-sized head on top of such a tiny body screams "created for strength."

It's simply genius. Think of it. A creature with a planet for a head placed on top of a blade of grass for a body. Then, to top it off, a righting reflex is placed in the head to FORCE the child to get strong enough to keep the head level with the horizon. If that doesn't scream strength, nothing does.

The righting reflex is a reflex that causes the head to become level with the horizon, which in turn causes the body to right its orientation to the head. In other words, the head is programmed to be on the horizon, and the body is programmed to follow and support the head.

This reflex initiates the next layer of strength that the diaphragm started- the center of strength wrapped around the epicenter of strength. I say this because the movements of the head are intimately connected to the body's core musculature. When the head and neck move into flexion, it causes the anterior chain to reflexively activate. When the head and neck move into extension, it causes the posterior chain to reflexively activate. In other words, head and neck flexion facilitates body flexion, and head and neck extension facilitates body extension.

Likewise, when the head and neck move into rotation, it facilitates the rotation of the torso by reflexively engaging the muscles that rotate the spine.

The righting reflex is initiated by the Vestibular System, which is also located in the child's Jupiter-sized head. The Vestibular System is the movement detection system and the sensory information collection system of the body. It detects all movement the body makes or all movement made upon the body, and it is also the collection hub for almost all incoming sensory information the body generates and receives. This is really the system that helps you be *you*.

The Vestibular System is an impressive work of art. It assists in building and protecting your brain, provides you with balance, coordination, control, and posture, and is interwoven with your other sensory systems like your visual and proprioception systems. Yes, that's right, the Vestibular System is the system of strength. If it is compromised, you CANNOT express strength.

A healthy vestibular system is essential for optimal strength expression and a happy life.

How do you keep your Vestibular System healthy? You move a lot. Throughout the day, intentionally challenge gravity and change body positions. This stimulates your vestibular system in so many different ways. It also lets your brain know that everything about your body is needed and wanted - the brain won't prune anything away that is needed and wanted. It only prunes away what is not being used, what is costing resources to be wasted.

A healthy vestibular system is essential for optimal strength expression and a happy life.

The other way to keep your Vestibular System healthy is to actually use your head. Instead of keeping your head fixed straight ahead or hanging down looking at an electronic device, you need to move it often, looking left and right, up and down, and you should return it level with the horizon every chance you get. That's where it wants to be anyway; that is where the righting reflex forced you to go as a child.

This also means moving your eyeballs through their full range of motion. The eyes are wired to lead the head, and the head is wired to lead the body. This means the eyes lead the body, too. If they are not being used and moved through their full range of motion often, the body will be missing out on vital information that it looks for to establish its foundation of reflexive strength.

This means the movement of your eyes can greatly affect your ability to express your full strength potential. Don't overthink this; just use your eyes and head often throughout the day. You'll feel better and be stronger. Period.

Gait, the Full Swing of Things

Beyond having an overly sized large head at birth, the human body has some other interesting design characteristics. It is not only shaped like a big, flexible X, but it is actually tied together and wired together by a series of X's. It is literally layers upon layers of X's woven together - from the muscles to the joint connections, from the DNA helixes to the sheaths of fascia, you are a series of spirals and X's that are woven together to produce efficient elastic, powerful motion.

But you're also wired as an X; that is, the circuits (the nerves and the neural connections) in your nervous system are cross-wired. The right side of your brain controls the left side of your body, and the left side of your brain controls the right side of your body. The movement of the right side of your body builds and nourishes the left side of your brain, and the movement of the left side of your body builds and nourishes the right side of your brain. The movements of your body even create neural connections between the two halves of your brain.

We are literally wired to move for and by contra-lateral movement. And that's pretty wild. Only Nature can fathom the wisdom in that. I can only see that it's pretty awesome.

Anyway, we are an X that is built through layers and series of Xs, and it is the mechanical design of our X moving contra-laterally through our gait pattern that builds, strengthens, and keeps our brain and nervous system healthy.

If you're following me, I'm saying that walking makes us stronger and stronger still.

I know it's not the typical movement we think about when we think about strength training, though its popularity in the strength world seems to be catching on a bit. But real walking, with all four limbs in full, uninhibited swing, is strength in motion. Walking with all four limbs takes advantage of our elastic recoil, made possible by the series of Xs that envelop our torso. Walking also keeps the brain healthy and the body reflexively tied together.

We have a self-perpetuating design for strength. The gait pattern builds an efficient and healthy nervous system that feels connected and safe. This safe nervous system, in turn, optimizes the output or performance of the body, allowing for strength to ooze out of every movement.

A body that crawls, walks, and runs well is a body that can produce speed, force, and power. It's also a body with rhythm, ease, coordination, balance, optimal posture, and grace.

Don't miss this. It is the full and free swing of each limb (there are four) in a coordinated rhythm with one another that builds and allows strength to express itself. Walking with only the legs, not allowing the shoulders to mirror them, does not take full advantage of the design of our nervous system. It "short changes" the information going to the brain and misses out on keeping all areas of the brain healthy. This type of walking is incomplete, just as partially using the diaphragm to breathe is incomplete.

Incomplete information will cause the brain to restrict our access to our full-strength expression because incomplete information is not "safe" information. It also literally weakens or undermines the full, possible neural net connections between the left and right hemispheres of the brain. Not only can this lead to inhibited expression of strength, but it can also lead to inhibited creativity and a dampened ability to focus, think, and remember.

In other words, not engaging in our full gait pattern can weaken all of us - body, mind, and soul.

I should point out that we have a more than wonderful design. There are some people who can't freely use all four limbs due to accidents, defects, traumas, and other issues. There are "backups" in the body. If we can cross the midline with parts of our body, we can activate and connect both hemispheres of our brain together. It may not be "optimal," but it is optimal as long as we use what we have to our fullest ability. Crossing midline with the limbs we have, or the other movers we have like our tongue, eyeballs, neck, and pelvis - these all take advantage of our cross-wiring connections and strengthen our nervous system.

The lesson here is really to move everything you have often. Even if you can't walk, move what you can through a full range of motion from left to right and from right to left. It helps remove inhibitions, and it creates strength.

You are an X. So be an X. Cross midline with your members often. Crawl, walk, skip, march, and run with all four limbs in beautiful, free, coordinated movement with one another often.

To review, here are the pillars and layers of strength for the human body:

1. Breathe with an uninhibited diaphragm.
2. Activate your vestibular system through movement and have full control of your head.
3. Engage in your full gait pattern.

Remember, while these three things do knit together and strengthen the body, they don't stop there. They also knit together all of you. Your thoughts and emotions are also strengthened by how you breathe and move. Everything about you is connected; you are whole. If your body is strong and healthy, your mind and emotions will also benefit from strength.

The Mind

"Free your mind and the rest will follow."
- Free Your Mind, En Vogue

You are whole indeed, and everything affects everything. This means your mind and thoughts affect your body and how it moves and feels. I mentioned this above, but the body follows the head. This is true physically and mentally. Where the thoughts go, the body will follow.

Did you know that you've never had a thought that your body was unaware of? Think about that. You cannot hide your thoughts from your body. Every thought you've ever had and will have is information that your brain is filtering to determine its safety and comfort level. But it's bigger than that, too. Your thoughts are essentially programs, and your body is essentially the hardware they program.

You've never had a thought that your body was unaware of.

This means you need to be aware of how you think when it comes to expressing your strength. You also need to be aware of how you think about what you think. Your attention or focus intensifies your thoughts. Attention adds weight to your thoughts. If you are thinking "safe," positive, light thoughts and focused on those thoughts, your brain will give you more access to your strength. If you think "not safe," negative, fearful thoughts, and you are focused on those thoughts, your brain will inhibit or govern your strength.

Thoughts are tricky. We can control them, the conscious ones. But the unconscious ones, sometimes they just happen. They may just happen because of our emotions or thought patterns, but sometimes, thoughts pop up uninvited. Sometimes, these uninvited thoughts can be so strange they actually concern us about our own mental health. "Dark" thoughts can just pop into our heads seemingly out of nowhere. They are clearly "not safe" thoughts, and they can just happen no matter how much we don't want them to happen.

This is one reason we need to be aware of our thoughts and the attention we give them. How and what we think about our thoughts gives them the power to either build us up or tear us down. We want to create safe information in our brains to allow our strength to flourish. This means we may need to let those unwanted thoughts slip through our minds without placing any weight on them through hyper-focus.

If it helps, there is a secret about these unwanted thoughts: they don't mean anything. Unwanted thoughts don't mean anything other than the meaning you give them. Sometimes, thoughts do just happen. Let them happen. Don't marinate on them or try to analyze them. Yes, they may be fearful thoughts but don't continue to think about them. You can be aware of them, acknowledge them, laugh at them, think them interesting and odd, but let them pass.

If you let those uninvited thoughts disturb you, if you hold on to them and rehearse them, if you ponder them, they will become toxic, negative information that will, in turn, negatively affect your entire body.

But if you let them go and place no weight on them whatsoever, they become a weak, passing threat at best. Your brain won't overly concern itself with them. They become nothing more than a passing cloud.

This takes practice, by the way. It's just like strength training. Wait, this is strength training - for your mind and soul. Practicing letting go of thoughts that could otherwise be harmful and destructive is a form of strength training. With time and practice, you learn to let thoughts just happen without a care about them. Soon, you find that those wild thoughts may happen less and less. Whether they lessen or not doesn't matter; how you allow them to pass matters.

If you should have any unwanted thoughts, practice saying this to yourself (give yourself a new thought to rehearse):

"This thought doesn't mean anything."

Say it. Believe it. Move on.

Even if you have to say it 1000 times, say it. That builds strength in your brain through repetition. It's also 1000 repetitions of a non-threatening thought. When you can let the weight of an unwanted thought pass through you, you will actually feel lighter and freer, as if a weight was removed from your body. And it has been.

But what about the thoughts you can control?

Work them to your advantage. Remember, your thoughts are programs. The unwanted thoughts are programs, too, but by letting them pass, they are brief, weak programs. But the thoughts that you consciously choose to create can be powerful programs. You can proactively create thoughts to program your body for health and strength.

Thinking positive, happy, affirming thoughts. Purposefully and intentionally focusing on something that brings you joy or something that you want (like strength) actually sends "safe" information to your brain that allows you to move and feel better. The more you focus on these thoughts, this positive information, the stronger you make the neural connections necessary to create and rehearse these thoughts.

You can literally wire your brain with positive thoughts and messages that can help to remove limitations from your mind and body. In other words, you can mentally rehearse yourself to be strong inside and out.

If this sounds crazy, be your own scientist and experiment and experience this for yourself.

Mentally say to yourself, "I am weak and afraid," a few times, then try to touch your toes or perform a deep squat. Notice how that felt.

Now, mentally say to yourself, "I am strong and courageous," a few times, then try to touch your toes or perform a deep squat. Notice how that felt.

Did you notice a qualitative difference between the two rehearsed thoughts? You likely noticed how your movements changed in ease, depth, and fluidity within seconds. Your thoughts can program your body at the speed of your nervous system. If a new thought can alter how your body moves, what do you think a rehearsed thought can do to your body's ability to express itself?

Don't miss the good news here though: A new thought can instantly change how your body feels and moves.

The point is your thoughts matter. They are real sources of information that influence how your body performs and functions. Thoughts are not just words, though; your imagination and your expectations are all thoughts. And as far as your body is concerned, they are real. Whatever you rehearse in your head is real to your body. Your nervous system will respond to your creative power, and the results will align with the safety and freedom of those thoughts.

For what it's worth, this is why Grandma can pick up a car from her grandbaby. She isn't thinking she can't do it. She is acting to do it. She is expecting to do it because she has to do it. There is no other alternative. Her expectation is to save her grandchild. She only knows how to move that car. And her nervous system only knows that she can move that car. It is not inhibited by her doubts or her fears. It is uninhibited by her expectation that she can move that car. Naturally, she doesn't have time to think about all of this; she just acts. But it is her actions that tell you what she truly believes. And it is her body that shows you.

Anyway, we need to strengthen and train our thoughts. We must mind the programs we create because our bodies will follow whatever we rehearse in our heads and hearts.

A simple way to do this would be to practice a mantra throughout the day, at a set time, or when a troubling thought or event happens.

Personally, I'm pretty sure this is how I get through life. I rehearse and marinate on thoughts and scriptures that bring me comfort and strength.

I hope it helps; some have gotten me through some tough times, including:

"Those who trust in the Lord shall have their strength renewed. They shall rise up on wings like an eagle. They shall run and not grow weary. They shall walk and not faint." Isaiah 40:31, with liberties

"Have I not told you? Be strong and courageous. Do not be afraid, and don't be discouraged, for I am with you wherever you go." Joshua 1:9, with liberties

"Don't be afraid. I am with you."

"I can do all things through Christ which strengthens me." Philippians 4:13

"I can do all things…"

"This, too, shall pass."

"And this is the secret: Christ is in you." Colossians 1:27

This may be a disturbing look into my psyche, but I have always found comfort in leaning on something bigger and stronger than me. And this is strengthening - for me.

If I might, let me tell you a story where this has really saved me - twice.

My wife and I were born 10 days apart. *We didn't know each other then; I'm just setting the story up.*

For our 30th birthday, we decided to have a huge joint celebration. We rented a limousine, got all our friends together, and tore up Raleigh, NC. It was an amazing night, full of amazing food, moments, laughter, and memories.

The next day started the same. We both woke up early and refreshed; we both felt amazing. We made plans to have our favorite pizza delivered for lunch. My wife told me she would go sit in the tub until the pizza came. When the pizza came, my wife called me into the bathroom. She didn't feel good. She didn't look good either. I had to pick her up from the tub and carry her to our bedroom. We ended up taking her to the hospital, where she stayed for almost a month.

Neither one of us saw this coming. We went from Heaven to Hell in less than a full day. My wife was sick, and the doctors didn't really know what to do at the time. The doctors eventually discovered she had a rare bacterial infection in one of her lungs; she had apparently gotten it from a construction site she was working on. The ultimate solution that ended up saving her life was removing the lower lobe of her left lung.

To say I was scared is an understatement. It's actually really hard to describe everything I was feeling. We had two toddlers, one and two years old, two beautiful babies. I was torn between spending days and nights at the hospital and making several trips back and forth to home to see my kids. It all just really sucked. I kept my Bible with me at the hospital. For some reason, Isaiah 43 found me. It seems like I read it 1000 times, if not more. That verse guided me through what we were experiencing; it strengthened me. It gave me a way to keep picking my head up when all I wanted to do was cry. It rescued me from the "What Ifs" that kept creeping up, and it gave me hope.

I'll share the verses that saved me:

"Don't be afraid. I have rescued you. I have called you by your name. You are Mine.

When you pass through the waters, I will be with you. When you go through the rivers of difficulty, you will not drown. When you walk through the fire, you will not be burned. Nor shall the flame scorch you." - Isaiah 43:1-2

Those words were a lifeline to me in some of my darkest hours. I needed Something bigger than me, and our situation and these words provided that. They kept stoking my strength and allowed me to support my wife unwaveringly when she needed something bigger than herself.

As I said, these words saved me twice. I will tell you the next story just for fun. It's amazing how things happen sometimes.

In 2019, my two beautiful babies had grown and were in High School. They both went on a trip to the Bahamas with our Church. While they were gone, my wife and I decided to go celebrate our 22nd wedding anniversary in Wilmington, NC. We were lounging by the pool when my wife got a phone call from a chaperone of the Bahamas trip. My oldest son had apparently jumped off a cliff into the ocean and had gotten injured. He was being airlifted in a small plane to a hospital in Nassau.

I'm sure I don't have to tell you this, but we were freaking the @$%# out. We didn't know if he hit his head, broke something, or if... We knew he was alive, and we knew we had to get to the Bahamas yesterday.

As it turned out, no emergency flights leaving in NC would take us to the Bahamas that day. So, while we were waiting for a 5:00 AM flight the next morning, my wife and I went for a walk to calm our nerves. We were a hot mess, I won't lie.

While we were walking, the chaperone called my wife when my son arrived at the hospital in Nassau. She had stayed with him the whole time. For some reason, she mentioned that my son's nurse had a tattoo on her arm that simply said "Isaiah 43:1." My wife asked me what that meant, and all I could do was laugh. The verse rescued me so many times while she was in the hospital all those years before. Right then, at that moment, I knew everything would be OK. I couldn't get to my son. I didn't know what was really wrong or going on. I was helpless, and I felt useless. But in an instant, Isaiah 43:1 ignited my strength, and it sustained me all the way to the Bahamas.

Words, mantras, phrases, and verses can strengthen you when you need to be strengthened. They can push out the fear just long enough to let your strength rise from within you when facing your toughest challenges. I've experienced this so many times.

Again, you don't have to recite verses. You can marinate on what you know to be true and what you want to be true. Simple, true statements like this can carry you through life's trials and events:

"I can do this."

"I am strong."

"I am enough."

These are not only "safe" messages to your brain; they are strength messages for your brain. They can lift inhibitions from your mind and body, allowing your strength to flow in a greater abundance than it otherwise would.

The point is that your thoughts influence your emotions and your body. They do so in accordance with the weight you allow them to have. They are messengers of safety, and some messages can be heavier than others.

Be mindful of the thoughts you keep and what thoughts you try to hold. Let nonsensical, uninvited thoughts pass through you. Don't grab hold of them. They don't mean anything unless you focus on them. Once they have your focus, they have you.

And stack the deck in your favor. Marinate on and rehearse affirming thoughts of strength, power, and joy. The more you rehearse them, the stronger you make them, making them more real. They are true, but they become real when you experience them.

Keep this in mind when you are struggling with emotions as well. If you are sad, you will likely have a dampener on your strength and performance. If you are bitter, cynical, or apathetic, this will likely inhibit your strength. Anger, though it is negative energy, is actually a higher emotion than fear, depression, and apathy. It may actually bolster your strength, as anger is often accompanied by confidence and courage to act. Anger can grant access to strength depending on who you are and where you are coming from.

And Happiness is extremely "safe." If you are happy, everything you move will be freer, more graceful, and more powerful. Happiness invigorates your expression suit (your body). So does the excitement of love. You know this is so. Nothing invigorates you like that first kiss from that special person you're head over heels for. That first kiss will make you feel like Superman or Wonder Woman. It removes all your inhibitions.

You can't have that first kiss every day, but even its memory can bolster you. After all, a memory is nothing more than a practiced or rehearsed thought. And that's the point; practice your thoughts - the useful ones.

Your mind is a doorway to your strength on all levels. A courageous mind than can ("I can"), can. A fearful, worrisome mind that can't, cannot. Your mind grants or blocks access to your strength. It's best to have a courageous mind that can. You can build a courageous mind through practice.

Don't let thoughts of fear and darkness sabotage your strength. They will dim your life in all other areas as well. Dwelling on fear, worries, and negativity is also a form of practice. Remember, our nervous system likes to be efficient. If we dwell on something, we are rehearsing and practicing it. Whatever we practice, we strengthen. If we practice negativity, we strengthen its effects and etch them into our nervous system. It's like eating kryptonite on purpose. It's toxic, and it robs us of our strength.

There is a wellspring of strength within you. The goal is to allow it to flow out of you unencumbered. You can do this by sending a continual, clear message of safety to your brain by moving the way you were designed to move and using your mind rather than allowing your mind to use you.

Just don't forget, your body is an expression suit. It will express your thoughts, your emotions, and your beliefs.

The Economics of Strength

"Strength training is simply asking your body for what you want."
- me

The nervous system is actually designed for strength. It works to create strong neural pathways that require very little energy to maintain. It also works to deconstruct or prune away pathways that are not needed, pathways that have an energy cost with no return.

"Use it or lose it," you've heard this a thousand times. It is the principle of neural pruning. Again, this can also be seen as the "Use it to Keep it" principle; you keep what you use through movement, thought, and habits. The more you use it, the deeper you entrench it. The less you use it, the more you erode it.

This is one of the miracles of the body; the nervous system is malleable and adaptable. It's plastic and never etched in stone. This means you have much " say " about what gets programmed into your nervous system. In fact, you get to essentially create your nervous system through the choices and actions you make on a routine basis.

If you have a habit or something you want to be free from, you can potentially erase it from your nervous system or replace it by creating new neural pathways. You could weaken the bad habit and try to erase it through disuse, or you could try to weaken it and replace it through investing in the "use" of other patterns, thoughts, and habits. The trick is to do something long enough to establish it and etch it into your nervous system or to abstain from something long enough to weaken it and dissolve it from your nervous system.

It sounds really simple, right? You can construct the nervous system you want. The rub is that this may not be so easy. It can be hard to break or erase neural connections (habits) that you want to break. This is because those neural patterns are very strong patterns - they've been entrenched into your nervous system by the lifestyle you've been living.

Bad habits are a representation of strong neural pathways, pathways that are so powerful they are like tractor beams that suck you into doing them. You almost can't not do them because their neural wiring is so strong. It takes very deliberate thought and action to create the desired change in your nervous system. But it can be done because you are a creator. You can create the changes you want to experience. All you have to do is live the life you want and express your strength by aligning your thoughts, emotions, and actions in the direction you want to go.

This is the economics of your nervous system. If you create a demand, your nervous system will gather up its resources and create the supply. Your nervous system will not waste resources if you don't demand anything. It will conserve them instead, and there will be no supply to match the demand that is not created.

If you create a demand, your nervous system will gather up its resources and create the supply.

In other words, you won't be an Olympic Sprinter if you've never asked your body to sprint. If all you do is sit in chairs, you're essentially asking your body not to be good at walking and running, but you are asking your body to be good at sitting in a chair.

My point is that your nervous system will give you what you ask it for, and the way to ask for things is through intention, repetitive use, and challenge. In other words, show up often and do the things you want to be good at. You can literally wire your nervous system to allow you to do the things you want to do. This includes expressing your strength potential.

One way to remove the inhibitions of strength is to simply move often in your designed movement patterns; these are the patterns that are hardwired into your nervous system. Remember the three movement pillars from earlier? We want to be experts at these three things:

1. Breathe properly with the diaphragm
2. Activate the vestibular system regularly
3. Engage in our contra-lateral gait pattern

These three things and all the neural connections that fire to make these three things happen are the foundation of every movement you can make. If you move well in these designed patterns often, you keep all the neural connections of those patterns "sharp" and entrenched. You are also creating a foundation of strength from which all other movements, thoughts, and emotions are connected.

On top of this foundation, the desired repetitive actions and thoughts you make build and entrench more neural networks. These networks are continually strengthened through use. They are also protected because a healthy brain will not prune away the continually used patterns.

Also, did you ever notice how the forbidden fruit was found on the Tree of The Knowledge of Good and Evil in the Story of

Creation? Both Good and Evil came from the same tree. Your nervous system is a tree of sorts. All the "good" you want can be found and built in it. But so can all the "bad." The fruit we produce (the outcomes of our expressions) comes from the strong neural connections that we create. An unwanted or "bad" habit also represents strong neural connections. Your nervous system is designed for strength - strength that bears the good or the bad. The fruit it bears (desired or undesired) results from your created strength.

If you're not following me, here's the point: You can cultivate and prune your neural tree to bear the fruits you want to bear. And that is AWE-some.

BEING STRONG

"Strength is as strength does."
- modified from Forrest Gump

As mentioned earlier, strength has layers. There is the strength we are programmed to express through our movement design, and there is the strength we are created to build through the plasticity of our nervous system. We can remove neural inhibitions and express our strength potential through moving and being as we are designed. While we each have the hidden strength of the heroic grandma saving her baby, we don't usually have full access to that strength without a catalyst that helps remove our inhibitions. Typically, we have many catalysts (stressors) that actually bury our strength and dampen our potential.

This is why taking advantage of our neural plasticity to practice and refine the strength we want to express is also a good idea. By showing up and practicing strength, practicing movements with and without extra load, we can make our nervous systems very efficient and "comfortable" with these practiced movements.

Remember, what we do on a regular basis, we get ridiculously good at. This is the SAID principle in action: we adapt to what we do. This is why I LOVE Dan John's Easy Strength training protocol. You show up daily and practice five movements for ten reps each. You use your body every day, establish strong, efficient neural pathways for those movements and you literally etch strength into your nervous system. It's brilliant.

This is my oversimplification of Easy Strength. There is much more to it as Dan presents it. I encourage you to check out his book, *The Easy Strength Omnibook*. It is a phenomenal resource for practicing the art of strength.

Taking the baton from Dan, if we want our strength to be uninhibited in the real world, it is a good idea to practice movements that are similar to the movements you would want and need to make in the real world.

Practicing the push, the pull, the squat, the hinge, the throw, the carry, and our gait patterns are worthy movements to train to refine, harness, and express our strength. These are also the same movements we would each be making daily and throughout the day if we lived a thousand years ago.

I love our modern world; I do. With the advances in technology, we are a blessed generation. But with all the gifts of our modern world, there is also a major setback; it circumvents our design by removing our need to move. Through our technology and advancements, we have separated ourselves from the world. This is the main reason why having a strength practice is so valuable; it is both a solution and a substitution.

Good strength training honors our design by causing us to "mimic" the movements we are designed to make when we are actually a part of the world around us. And make no mistake, we are meant to be a contributing part of the world and move in the world. That, too, is part of our design.

But speaking of design, if we are designed to push, pull, squat, hinge, carry, and travel, these are absolutely the things we need to be doing in some fashion on a daily basis. The best way to use a tool is in how it was intended to be used.

Your body was intended and designed to be used and moved daily. This is where strength is found, in engaging and being in our design. In the following section, I offer some training routines you can use to find your strength.

Gaining Access to Strength

Below, I share several routines designed to help you gain access to your strength. These routines are by no means the only ways that work to build strength. But they are somewhat gentle ways that honor your body's design in the pursuit of optimal strength expression.

What I mean is that they take advantage of your neurology. They require showing up and engaging often. That's the key to unlocking your strength. Strength is found in the doing.

Yes, you could train like a powerlifter or a cross-fitter. There's nothing wrong with that. But if you're doing these things in the absence of a solid foundation of reflexive strength or on top of a nervous system that is highly guarded and reserved, you will find roadblocks and limitations to your strength. This is why I think Pressing RESET is really non-negotiable in any movement practice; it grants access to your body's abilities.

So you can go very heavy if you want to. But do you need to? Will deadlifting 500 pounds make your life better? Maybe, but maybe not. It could etch in one movement pattern that you're really good at (the deadlift itself) and perhaps impede other movement patterns that you want to be good at (like walking up and down stairs).

There is also another cost to consider. Heavy loads can end up being too heavy for what is optimal. Just because you can squat 600 pounds doesn't mean it's good for you to do so on a regular basis. The body does adapt to what it does unless what it does overrides what the body can handle. If the stress is higher than the stress needed for an optimal growth and recovery response, the stress will ultimately lead to breakdown and injury. That means, in the long term, the big picture of health and strength, being able to do 200 bodyweight squats may be more beneficial than doing one 600-pound barbell squat.

I guess my point is, again, you have all the strength you'll ever need in your body. You are strong enough. You need access to your strength, which is granted through a nervous system that feels safe. It is not granted by a nervous system that is constantly over-stressed and threatened. It's not about how much weight you can lift. It's about how well you can move.

The programs below offer ways to access your strength through learning how to move very well with and without manageable loads. The better you move, the better you feel. The better you feel, the stronger you are. Remember, it feels good to feel strong. But it feels even better to KNOW you are strong.

You are strong right now.

There, don't you feel better?

THE ROUTINES OF ENGAGEMENT

"Make it so."
- Jean-Luc Picard, Star Trek the Next Generation

As one size does not fit all in all things in life. The following routines and examples are just some of the ways I've found useful in gaining access to my strength. Some of these routines may work very well for you, others not so much.

We all have different lives, body proportions, environments, time demands, preferences, abilities, resources, etc. It would stand to reason that there will be many different ways we can get from A to Z. Honestly, I wanted to write "skin a cat" instead of "get from A to Z," but I didn't know if that was acceptable. Navigating an ever-changing world is challenging!

That's another reason for the following routines: things change. You change. Your life will go through seasons. There may be seasons in your life where all you can do is Press RESET for 10 minutes in the morning. That is okay. There may be other seasons in your life where you just want to pick up weight and move it around. That is okay. The routines below can be used with the varying seasons that happen both around you and in you.

Anyway, these routines are ways to take advantage of your nervous system's economics, movement patterns, and design. This is not by any means an exhaustive list or a "This is the way" list of routines. You may not think much of these routines if you are a powerlifter. However, if you are a powerlifter, getting ridiculously good at owning the three pillars of human movement I discussed earlier is a great way to take your strength training and strength expression to new frontiers.

For the brave, I encourage you to test these routines. Experience them and discover how they make you feel. Determine for yourself if they grant you access to your strength and ability. Test them out and see if they enhance your resilience and your peace.

Press RESET

I know I just said one size doesn't fit all, but this one thing does. Press RESET on your body every day. The following movements honor the Three Pillars of Human Movement I mentioned earlier.

These movements make up a large part of the developmental sequence. They are the foundational movements for all the other movements you make. They also are the foundational movements for all the wonderful expressions you were designed to make.

I've written extensively about them in *Pressing Reset: Original Strength Reloaded*, so I will only present them here as "Do This Every Day."

In other words, this is your daily practice or your daily routine to ensure that you are always free to express yourself.

There are many ways to incorporate these five resets into your day. Still, I will give you only one simple example for simplicity's sake.

Every morning, do this:

Breathe x 2 minutes.

- Get in a comfortable position of your choice.
- Keep your lips shut, place your tongue on the roof of your mouth, and breathe in and out of your nose.
- Allow your belly and lower back to expand, thus filling your lungs up from the bottom to the top.

Nod and Rotate your head x 2 minutes

- Get in a comfortable position of your choice.
    - Varying positions have various advantages. Explore them all.
- Leading with your eyes, nod your head up and down as far as your neck will allow you to.
    - The eyes go up, the head goes up. The eyes go down, the head goes down.
    - Keep breathing as above.
    - Don't move into pain.
    - Do this for 1 minute.
- Leading with your eyes, rotate your head left and right as far as your neck will allow you to.
    - The eyes go right, the head goes right. The eyes go left, the head goes left.
    - Keep breathing as above.
    - Don't move into pain.
    - Do this for 1 minute.

Roll on the Floor x 2 minutes

- Lie on your back with your arms overhead.
- Keep your legs relaxed and free of any tension.
    - Pretend they are limp, wet noodles.
- Leading with your eyes and your head, take your right arm and reach across your body over your left hip.

- Allow your reach to simply pull your body all the way over until you are lying on your belly.
- You want your body to roll one vertebra at a time, piece by piece, fluidly like an ocean wave.
- Then, look right over your shoulder, take your right arm, and reach back across your body until you roll back to your back.
- Next, do the same with the left arm.
- Keep breathing as above.
- Work your upper body rolls from side to side and arm to arm for 1 minute.

- Then, Lie on your back with your arms overhead.
- Keep your arms and upper body relaxed and free of any tension.
- Pull your right knee up towards your chest and then reach across your body towards your right shoulder with your right foot as if you are trying to reach something.
  - Allow your reach to simply pull your body all the way over until you are lying on your belly.
  - Again, you want your body to roll one vertebra at a time, piece by piece, fluidly like an ocean wave.
- When you are on your belly, bend your right knee, reach your foot up towards the ceiling, and then across your body until the reach rolls you over to your back.
- Next, do the same with your left leg.
- Keep breathing as above.
- Work your lower body rolls from side to side and from leg to leg for 1 minute.

Rock on your hands and knees x 2 minutes

- Get on your hands and knees and keep your eyes and head level with the horizon.
  - Hold your head up so that you can see the world.
- Keep a "proud" chest or pretend to be a silverback gorilla.

- Rock your but back towards your feet as far as you can maintain this posture, and then rock back forward so that your weight shifts over your hands.
- Rock back and forth with your feet in plantar flexion (top of foot against floor, or laces down) x 1 minute
- Rock back and forth with your feet in dorsiflexion (ball of foot on floor) x 1 minute.
- Keep breathing as above.
- Don't let your head drop or your back round.

Crawl x 2 minutes

- Get on your hands and knees and keep your eyes and head level with the horizon.
  - Hold your head up so that you can see the world.
- Keep a "proud" chest or pretend to be a silverback gorilla.
- Crawl forward, backward, and/or sideways by moving opposite limbs together.
  - Your opposing limbs should move smoothly together, lifting and landing, at or near the same time.
- Keep breathing as above.
- Don't let your head drop or your back round.

These may be the most important movements you could ever do. Because of that, I'll provide some video links here so you can see them in action.

Breathing: https://youtu.be/DCAyHVhuPJE

Head Nods and Rotations: https://youtu.be/jWWOIi8_YqM

Rolling: https://youtu.be/IEtmbw9XdiI

Rocking: https://youtu.be/5e08_N8Ca7M

Crawling: https://youtu.be/kGIQ4szkb4c

The Daily 21's

I wrote extensively about the Daily 21's in my book, *Discovering You*. I'm including them here because they are simply wonderful in building a strong, efficient nervous system that will grant access to optimal strength expression.

The concept is you perform the following movements every day for 21 repetitions per day. These movements do not require equipment (except for the optional pull-up). They only require engagement. They are perfect for those who love calisthenics. There is no harm in doing both the RESETS that I listed above and these. In fact, that is a terrific daily training session.

The challenge in these movements will vary from person to person. For some, these may be quite difficult in the beginning. If that is the case, you can perform seven sets of three or break up the repetitions however you need to in order to reach your 21 reps. For others, these movements may be quite easy or eventually become easy. That is great! You can increase their difficulty and your effort by slowing them down and exploring them.

Don't try to blast through them to check them off. Learn to savor them and learn from them. There is gold to mine here.

If this is the route of strength training that you want to take, do these every day:

The Daily 21s for Strength and Wellbeing

- The Head and Leg Raise x 21 repetitions
- The Swinging Table Top x 21 repetitions
- The Waving Hindu Pushup x 21 repetitions
- The Elevated Roll Dance x 21 total rolls
- The Hindu Squat x 21 repetitions
- The Wave Squat x 21 repetitions

- The Track Starter x 21 repetitions per leg (42 total movements)
- Extra Credit:
  - o Pull-ups, Chin-ups, or Horizontal Rows x 21 total repetitions

To keep this book less than 500 pages, I'll simply include a video of these movements here: https://youtu.be/nXqAfHgDuj4

The Easy 21's

The Easy 21's are something I have enjoyed for quite some time. It is the love child of Dan John's Easy Strength and my Daily 21's. The idea is to perform 21 repetitions of the major human movements of pushing, pulling, hinging, and squatting daily. You can also add in accessory movements as you wish, like bicep curls or lateral raises. The movements can be done with a barbell, kettlebells, dumbbells, bodyweight, or the tools you choose.

You can stick with the same movements every day, or you can vary them daily. You can also vary how you get to 21 reps of each movement on any given day. You can perform sets of 11 and 10, 3 sets of 5 and one set of 6, 7 sets of 3 reps, 3 sets of 7 reps (I like this one), or 21 straight reps. Varying the sets and reps to a total of 21 daily helps with focus and practice. It allows you to learn from the movements. It also allows you to easily vary the loads or the intensity from day to day as you wish.

Speaking of the loads, light loads work here. The highest weight I've used on the barbell was 70% of my body weight. At

165 pounds, I never used more than 115 pounds. Often, I would vary my loads to between 50% and 70% of my body weight on any given day.

Of course, if the movement was a bodyweight movement like dips or chin-ups, naturally, that was my full bodyweight. But if you do this, you will find that your body weight starts to feel quite light and easily manageable in your calisthenics.

Here is the hard part of the Easy 21s: It's a very loose structure. It allows for freedom and exploration - two things that make people very uncomfortable. It's funny how we think we want freedom until we have it. What we want is comfort, not freedom. But that's too big for this book!

Anyway, there are no hard rules here. You get to pick the movements you want to do day in and day out. You get to choose the sets and reps that total 21 repetitions. You get to vary the loads as your whims dictate. The rule is that you show up every day. OK, you can take Sundays off, but you don't have to.

I cannot encapsulate all the ways you could set up your Easy 21s. So, I will simply show you my template or what I have enjoyed for about nine straight months. This will also give you an opportunity to see how I view "loose structure."

Oh yeah, on all days, begin your training practice by Pressing RESET for 10 minutes.

Mondays
115-pound barbell Complex of Power Cleans (hinge), Push-press (vertical push), and Front Squats, superset with Chin-ups (vertical pull).

- Power Clean x 7, Push-press x 7, Front Squat x 7, then put the bar down and perform Chin-ups x 7.
- Rest
- Repeat two more times.

Then,
- Bodyweight dips x 21
- Dumbbell curls x 21
- Hanging knee raises x 21
- Lateral shoulder raises x 21

Then,
- Carries (suitcase, overhead, etc) x 10 minutes

Tuesdays
Two 16K kettlebells Complex of Double Snatches (hinge), Double Press (vertical push), Double Front Squat

- Double Snatch x 7
- Double Press x 7
- Double Front Squat x 7
- Rest
- Repeat twice more.

Then,
- Chin-ups x 11, 10
- Bicep Curls x 11, 10
- Dips x 21
- Ab Wheel x 7, 7, 7
- Lateral Raises x 11, 10

Then,
- Crawl practice x 10 minutes (not continuous but broken up segments to allow practice and focus).

Wednesdays
95-pound barbell

- Power Snatch (hinge) x 6, 5, 5, 5
- Squat Thruster (squat and vertical push) x 6, 5, 5, 5

Then,
- Pull-ups x 6, 5, 5, 5
- Dips x 21
- Empty Barbell Biceps curls x 21

- Lateral Raises x 21
- Hanging Knee raises x 7, 7, 7

Then,

- Marching practice with Indian Clubs x 10 minutes

Thursdays

105-pound barbell
Chain of Power Clean, to Press, to Front Squat

- Power Clean x 1, Press x 1, Front Squat x 1 x 7 reps
- Rest
- Repeat for two more rounds.

Then,

- Chin-ups x 7, 7, 7
- Biceps Curls x 11, 10
- Dips x 21
- Lateral Raises x 11, 10
- Ab Wheel x 7, 7, 7

Then,

- Carries (suitcase, overhead, etc) x 10 minutes

Fridays

24K kettlebell

- Dead-hang Snatch (hinge) x 6r/6l, 5r/5l, 5r/5l, 5r/5l
- Side Press (vertical press) x 6r/6l, 5r/5l, 5r/5l, 5r/5l
- Split Stance Squat x 6r/6l, 5r/5l, 5r/5l, 5r/5l

Then,

- Chin-ups x 6, 5, 5, 5
- Dips x 21
- Biceps Curls x 11, 10
- Lateral Raises x 21
- Hanging Knee Raise x 6, 5, 5, 5

Then,

- Crawl Practice x 10 minutes

Saturdays
95-barbell

- Power Snatch x 7, 7, 7
- Clean and Jerk x 7, 7, 7
- Front Squat x 21

Then,

- Pull-up x 7, 7, 7
- Dips x 21
- Biceps Curl x 21
- Lateral Raise x 7, 7, 7
- Ab Wheel x 11, 10

Then,

- Marching practice with Indian Clubs x 10 minutes

That's what most of my weeks have looked like for nearly a year. You can see the loose structure in that Mondays and Thursdays, Tuesdays and Fridays, and Wednesdays and Saturdays are roughly the same. Inside each day, the sets and reps to reach 21 total reps varies. The complex and chain days obviously have another huge variable of time under tension, as the barbell is not released until all the numbers of the complex or chain have been reached.

Each day is concluded with a form of gait practice, such as carrying an object for time and distance, crawling, or marching. Every session started with Pressing RESET. Most of these routines would take me between 45 - 60 minutes.

All sessions were at a very relaxed pace. All sessions lent themselves to strength and well-being. I have felt very refreshed and strong for most of the year (I had a bout with Shingles, which slowed me down for three days).

Your Easy 21s practice can look any way you want it to. Just commit to showing up often. Try for 5 to 6 days a week, but also allow life to happen. Perform 21 reps of a push, pull, hinge, squat, and anything else you want to practice. For your loads, keep it simple and light. Use the load to facilitate concentration and proper contractions and movement. Play between 40 to 70% of your optimal or desired body weight. KEEP the loads light. Do the Dan John's Easy Strength program if you want to go heavy or heavier.

If you are so inclined, end your Easy 21's practice with a crawl or a carry. I'll talk more about crawls and carries in the next section. Just know they complete the movements we were designed to make daily.

If we recall the RPE scale, I mentioned at the beginning of the book, the Easy 21s probably dance in the realm of a 5 RPE. They will slowly nudge your 5 to a 3. So it is okay to up the load or the resistance when you feel like you need to be at a 5. But, in the spirit of practice, exploring your movements and learning from them is also okay. It's okay if your practice is only a 3 on the RPE scale on some days. If you are learning and enjoying your practice, let that be enough. After all, you are showing up every day, and that lets your body know that you want access to it, that you care for it, and that you respect it.

The Easy 21s work. It is a great way to build an efficient, strong nervous system that will give you access to your strength. It can also be a way to build aesthetically pleasing muscle - if you are patient and if you show up.

Super Simple Strength

There is another method I am rather fond of for building and maintaining strength. I call it the Super Simple Strength program. This is a program that I once wrote about on my blog. That particular blog generated some good discussions about strength training. In fact, it generated more discussion than almost any article I've written.

It overlaps much with the Easy 21's, but as the name suggests, this is still a lot simpler. Here is the gist of it.

In the Super Simple Strength program, all you do is "pick 2, then carry or crawl."

You pick two movements and superset them back and forth for ten to twenty minutes, getting in the work that you can WHILE maintaining NASAL BREATHING. This is a form of escalating density training. It's about getting work done in a specified amount of time.

After you complete this task, you perform a carry or a crawl for ten to twenty minutes. Again, you are trying to fill the ten to twenty minutes with as much "work" as possible while maintaining nasal breathing. If your mouth pops open, your body is telling you to rest. Honor it! When you can close your lips and recover, you resume the work.

This yields twenty total minutes of work that can be split up into two separate ten-minute segments to fit your day as you see fit.

There are two approaches to this method of escalating density training.

1. Let the clock run. If your mouth pops open, you should rest and recover until you can close it. Let the clock run while you rest. When the ten minutes expires, record how many rounds or how much work you completed. Every time you show up to train, you now have a metric that you can aim to meet or surpass.

2. Stop the clock. If your mouth pops open, rest and recover until you can close it, but STOP the clock while you are resting. When you can resume the movements with your lips closed, resume the clock. Here, you are training your movements for 10 minutes of total work completed.

When you have completed the 10 minutes of work, record how many minutes the session actually lasted. Every time you show up to train, you now have a metric that you can aim to beat. Eventually, you'll never need to stop the clock.

Anyway, you pick the two movements. I like sticking with the Fab Four: Push, Pull, Hinge, Squat - These can be bodyweight or loaded movements; it's up to you. But whatever you choose, remember you want to try to maintain a steady, constant work effort throughout, resting as little as you need to. So, the loads don't need to be very heavy; they just need to be challenging. Here, we are aiming for an RPE of 7 or 8!

Let's imagine that you chose the bodyweight squat for 10 reps and the pushup for 5 reps. You can now superset them or stack them back and forth one after another, at a steady pace for ten to twenty minutes.

Then, or later that day, you might choose to perform a "Goblet Carry" (front-loaded carry chest high) for 10 minutes, or you may decide you want to backward leopard crawl for 10 to 20 minutes.

Note: The carries and crawls DO NOT have to be continuous, without rest, per se. You can structure them to have a built-in "rest." For example, You may have 20 yards of real estate and a 50-pound kettlebell. You could perform 10 minutes of suitcase carries by picking the bell up in the right hand walking for 20 yards, and then putting it down. Turn around, pick it up in the left hand, and walk back the 20 yards. You put it down on the ends and carry it in the middle. This gives you "rest" but allows you to maintain constant work simultaneously.

You can do the same thing with the crawls. You could leopard crawl for 20 yards, then stand up and walk back the 20 yards. Repeat this for 10 minutes. The walk back is the "rest," but it is also movement and an opportunity to train your gait pattern. This is an amazing life-changing drill, by the way. It GIVES so much more than it takes. I'll repeat this because it's so slippery you can miss it. Combining a crawl for a certain distance with a walk, a cross-crawl, a march, or a skip is a wonderful way to invigorate your body and soul. It's also a great Sunday afternoon movement session on its own:

Crawl for 20 yards, march back for 20 yards. Repeat for 20 minutes. You're welcome.

For what it's worth, when you choose carries, I like using loads of 20 - 30% of optimal body weight. It doesn't have to be heavy, but you want it heavy enough to elicit a wonderful reflexive response from the body.

Now, I know I said Pick 2, then crawl or carry, but not all movements fall into the categories of push, pull, hinge, and squat. Some movements, like the Turkish Getup, are in a different category. For more complicated, whole-body movements that require a great deal of focus, I like to keep them on their own for a specified amount of time. I guess that would be a Pick 1, huh? So, in the example of Turkish Getups, it would be to Practice the getups for 10 minutes, then crawl or carry for 10 minutes. But that is just my preference.

That's the Super Simple Strength program in a nutshell. You may think this is too simple or too light to build a strong and capable body. But the proof is in the doing. If you can churn steady work while nasal breathing for 10 or 20 minutes and then perform carries or crawls for 10 or 20 minutes while nasal breathing, you'll build a strong AND resilient body, inside and out.

Here is an example of what this may look like:

Start each day with 10 minutes of Pressing RESET.

Day 1: Superset Squats x 10 reps and Pushups x 5 reps for 10 minutes. Then perform Overhead Carries x 10 minutes.

Day 2: Superset Kettlebell Swings x 10 reps and Pull-ups x 3 reps for 10 minutes. Then Backward Leopard Crawl x 10 minutes.

Day 3: Practice Bodyweight Getups, or Formal Turkish Get-ups, for 10 minutes. (You choose the sets and reps. Just be smart.) Then perform Goblet Carries (carries with the load held at chest height) x 10 minutes.

Day 4: rest

Rinse and repeat with the same movements or similar movements, or mix them up.

Here is another example of what this could look like:

Start each day with 10 minutes of Pressing RESET.

Day 1: Superset Hindu Squats x 20 reps and Hindu Pushups x 10 reps for 20 minutes. Then perform Overhead Carries x 10 minutes.

Day 2: Superset Power Cleans x 3 reps and Pull-ups x 3 reps for 10 minutes. Then Backward Leopard Crawl x 20 minutes.

Day 3: Perform Bodyweight Getups, or Formal Turkish Get-ups, for 10 minutes. Then perform Kettlebell Swings x 10 minutes (you choose the reps). Then perform Goblet Carries x 10 minutes.

There are no hard rules. I did "Pick 2," even with the getup. Here, I gave the getup and the swings dedicated practice time.

Day 4: Farmers Carries and Backwards Crawl x 20 minutes.

- Farmers Carry two "heavy" kettlebells 20 yards. Put them down. Backward Leopard Crawl back to where you started. Stand up and walk back to the bells. Repeat the process for 20 minutes.
- Carry, crawl, walk, carry, crawl, walk...

- I described this one because this is one of my favorite drills. It feels amazing to do, and it's too good not to share.

Day 5: Rest

As I said above in the Daily 21s program, there is a lot of gold here to mine. It's found in the faithful doing, in showing up every day and practicing. I know this is super simple. And it works. This is also super malleable. You can increase the desired work time for one, both, or either section. You can Squat and Pull for 20 minutes instead of 10. You can crawl and skip for 15 minutes or 22 minutes. It's up to you how seasoned you are in your training and how much work you want to accomplish. But in the beginning, just start with 10 minutes of both. Happy mining!

Walk This Way

"But I would walk 500 miles, and I would walk 500 more just to be the man who walks a thousand miles to fall down at your door."
- I'm Gonna Be, The Proclaimers

If you've been paying attention, this book is about gaining access to the enormous amount of strength that is already inside of you. Because of that, I will remind you about the movement I wrote about earlier - walking.

Without strength training, strength practice, weight lifting, cross-fitting, or whatever, Walking is THE RESET that will grant you access to your strength. It is the secret sauce you want to add to your life.

Walking is THE RESET that will grant you access to your strength.

I know this is a leap of faith, so let me tell you about my leap of faith.

I had reached a point in my daily strength practice where I would leopard crawl for 20 straight minutes every day. I would get on my hands and feet, set my eyes and head on the horizon, lower my butt below my head, start my clock, and crawl with my lips shut until 20 minutes expired on the clock. Every. Single. Day. And you know what? 20 minutes was as easy as 2 minutes. I felt strong; my body was strong, and I knew it.

About a year into crawling every day, as always happens, my season started to change. I didn't want to become a slave to 20 minutes as it was so easy for my disciplined personality, and I was dealing with some stressful issues in my life. I needed to make a change in my training routine. I had been telling people in the Pressing RESET certifications that walking was the extension of crawling and that walking was intended to keep us strong; I knew that in my head, but I did not *know* that in my body. I had not given myself the opportunity to explore walking as a strength-enhancing movement.

So, I started walking as my "main form" of strength training. Along with that, I also decided not to crawl at all. This was a huge decision for me; you have to understand that up to this point, I had been enjoying the benefits of crawling for almost five years. I knew in both my mind and body that crawling made me Superman.

For an entire year, I walked for my strength training. Yes, I still Pressed RESET and enjoyed bodyweight movements like Hindu Squats and Pushups, but that's all I did. I did not lift weights, and I did not crawl. I would take two to three daily walks for 10 to 45 minutes at a time. Sometimes, I would walk holding Indian Clubs; sometimes, I would walk with a weighted backpack on my back, and sometimes I would just walk without anything at all.

When I wore a backpack, I would have about twenty-five pounds of sand in the backpack. I rarely went much heavier than that. Regardless of what tools I was walking with, I focused on my shoulder swing, breathing, and gaze every time I walked. In other words, I ensured my shoulders were swinging rhythmically with my hips, my lips were shut with my tongue on the roof of my mouth, and my eyes and head were nestled on the horizon.

This was my strength training. I was literally stepping out in faith to learn if what I thought I knew was really real. After a year of walking, with NO weight training and NO crawling, I developed a weird curiosity about performing the Turkish Getup with a barbell. If you've never done a Getup with a barbell, it is not only a feat of strength but a feat of control and mastery. You can have no weak links in the chain of your body when performing a barbell Getup, especially a heavy barbell Getup.

This was a weird curiosity because, at this point, I had not been practicing the Turkish Getup for about two years. I put two 10-pound plates on a 45-pound barbell and easily performed a Getup on each side. It was easy and nice, so I made the barbell weigh 100 pounds. I easily performed a Getup on both sides with the 100-pound barbell.

Then, I had a weird thought from deep within me; it was almost like a whisper, "I bet you can do 135 pounds." The thought of this was both crazy and exhilarating at the same time. I had a weird sense of excitement, and now my curiosity begged me to find out.

So, I put two 45-pound plates on the barbell. I laid down, grabbed the barbell, pressed it up over my body, held it with one hand, and then stood up, holding it over my head. I then laid down with the barbell, AMAZED, switched hands and did it AGAIN with my left hand. Talk about proof in the pudding! I couldn't even believe it. This is just not a normal feat of strength! I only weighed 160 pounds and had just performed a Turkish Getup with 135 pounds once in BOTH hands. This displayed Super-Strength, the strength inside me waiting to be tapped into.

Here is the part of my story that gets a little weird. I heard a "whisper" telling me I could do this. Because of this whisper, I cannot tell you that walking is THE reason I was able to perform this Getup with 135 pounds. Because of the whisper, I must tell you that I think God filled me with the whisper and the strength to perform this unusual feat.

Regardless of what you or I believe in this matter, I can tell you that for a year, I did not crawl and for a year, I did not lift weights, or practice performing getups. I can tell you that I walked for the majority of my strength training for a year. But again, to be clear, I had a nudge and a whisper that led me to experience that Getup, so I can't confidently tell you that the walking allowed me the strength to perform that feat.

I know it's a crazy story; honestly, it's probably hard to believe. But just in case it helps, I actually videotaped that Getup.

Here it is: 135-Pound Get-up on Both Sides
https://youtu.be/IpZARHSBN6I

The point to all of this is, don't dismiss the power of walking. It takes the baton from crawling and continues perpetuating the miracles of our design to be a strong, capable, and powerful force throughout our entire lifetime.

Walking is the "vehicle" of our strength.

THE PURPOSE OF STRENGTH

"There is no greater strength than to lay down one's life for one's friends."
- John 15:13, NLT modified by me

We are designed to be strong, capable, and a powerful force throughout our lives. While this is not the message the world is telling you, this is the message that your very design is screaming. And this is a message that is worth screaming from the rooftops.

We are meant to live a life of strength.

Everything about our design points to this. And because of this, because we are designed to be strong, there must be a reason. After all, everything in nature has a purpose.

Why is the human born so helpless?

So it can develop strength and tenacity.

Why are humans more capable of thought and emotion than all other animals?

So it can harness, focus, and refine its strength and put it to good use.

What is the purpose of our strength?

To give it away.

This is why you were meant to be strong. This is why your body has all the strength in it you could ever need. We are meant to offer our strength to others. This is what Grandma does when she lifts the car off her precious grandchild. She gives herself away.

You've probably heard this, "Strength has a greater purpose." The purpose of strength is to serve others. To lift others. To love others.

Consider this. It is hard to love others, let alone serve others in our moments of weakness. When we are weak, when we feel weak, we are insecure, we are fearful, we become thoughtless, and we become selfish. In our weakness, we only seek to survive.

The purpose of strength is to serve others.

But when we are strong and know we are strong, we are confident, courageous, thoughtful, loving, giving, and generous. In our strength, we effortlessly thrive.

It is straightforward to give yourself to another and love others when you know you are strong. It is also hard to see another when consumed with your weaknesses and limitations. If you look at the totality of our design as humans, you can easily see a few things.

- We are made to move well and be strong throughout our lifetime.
- We are made for social interaction and cooperation.

- We are meant to be the stewards and caretakers of the
  entire world, including all its people, life forms, and
  resources.

We cannot do ANY of these things in weakness and the
self-centeredness that comes with it. We are literally designed for
strength, and it is our strength that enables us to Love. Love is an
extension of unabated strength.

Can you see this?

If we are meant to be strong, we are meant to love.

If we can gain access to all the strength that is inside of us,
we can gain more access to all the love that is inside of us as
well. If we become strong enough to forget about ourselves, we'll
be strong enough to give ourselves away. This is the purpose of
strength. And this is why you owe it to yourself and the entire
world to embark on a daily/almost daily strength practice.

This practice can be both physical and mental. It can be
movement-based and thought-based. There is no separation
between the mind and body. If we can experience physical
strength, we can know mental strength and vice-versa. And we
can also learn to rely on the strength that comes from Whispers.

True strength doesn't come from us; it comes through us. I can
write this to you today because I have experienced the Strength
that has come through me, both physically and spiritually. I was
not strong enough on my own to make it through my wife's
hospitalization. I was not strong enough on my own to not lose
myself when my son was injured. And I cannot tell you that it was
my strength that allowed me to perform the 135-pound Getup;
logically, that should not have happened. But what I can tell you,
along with the strength that was put in me, is that there is a
Greater Strength that comes through me, and that comes through
for me.

I am telling you this because it is also a great reminder to me. If we are designed to be strong and if strength is love, then we must be designed. Our Designer is Love. And for some reason, a reason I just can't figure out, Love wants to move through us.

There is no greater love than to lay down one's life for one's friends. In other words, there is no greater Strength than this. That is our purpose. Love, Strength, wants to move through us and be poured out from us. This is a strength that knows no limits.

So there it is. We are made for Strength.

I must tell you that I did not intend to end the book this way. I'm not sure how I intended to end it, but at this point, I'm just following a Whisper.

If you're unsure about what I'm saying in this last part or it's just not for you, that's ok. You're still designed to have access to your strength. Just engage in your design. Explore the routines in this book. Press RESET every day. Go for walks. Know that you are designed and meant to be strong. This is how you discover and reveal the strength that is in you. And if you engage in your design long enough and learn from it, you may even discover the Strength that wants to move through you.

"...I am fearfully and wonderfully made;
Marvelous are Your works,
And that my soul knows very well."
- Psalm 139:14

ABOUT THE AUTHOR

Tim is a movement education expert who works as an author, speaker, teacher, and trainer. His motto is "It feels good to feel good." He enjoys helping people learn how to feel great in their bodies. Tim is the creator of the Original Strength System, a program designed to restore a person's natural movement patterns.

He is enthusiastic about promoting health and wholeness and focuses on the whole person, including their body, mind, and spirit. Tim uses movement, humor, and an invitation to experience the wonder of your own body to teach this wholeness.

Tim has authored several books, including Pressing Reset: Original Strength Reloaded, The Becoming Bulletproof Project, Habitual Strength, Discovering You, and Be Naked. He has been featured in various news broadcasts and publications and presented his Original Strength System around the world.

Printed in the USA
CPSIA information can be obtained
at www.ICGtesting.com
CBHW071935120324
5272CB00009B/123